Chair Massage

The Complete Guide To Chair Massage Guide: Understanding The Tradition, Technique, And Transformative Healing

BANABAS WISDOM

Contents

Introductory

A chair massage is a specific category of massage in which the recipient remains seated on a chair that has been ergonomically designed for that purpose. In contrast to a full-body massage, this specific form of massage generally lasts for a reduced period of time and concentrates on the upper body, specifically the neck, shoulders, back, and arms.

The massage chair is portable and provides a relaxed, supported position for the recipient to recline while receiving the massage. The massage therapist can then address tension and stress in the targeted areas through the application of various massage techniques, including kneading, compression, and percussion. In locations where a complete massage table might be impractical, such as airports, offices, or public events, chair massages are frequently administered.

As a result of their portability and ability to induce relaxation and alleviate muscle tension rapidly, chair massages are prevalent in settings where individuals may lack the time for an extended massage session.

They can serve as an advantageous alternative for expeditiously reducing tension and enhancing overall wellness.

CHAPTER ONE
The Advantages Of Chair Massage

The numerous advantages that chair massages provide make them a popular option in a variety of contexts. The following are several potential advantages:

• Chair massages are portable and do not necessitate the removal of clothing by the recipient. Such environments as workplaces, public spaces, events, or offices, where a comprehensive massage may be impractical, can benefit from their convenience.

• Time-Saving: Chair massages are generally less time-consuming than conventional full-body massages, rendering them an advantageous choice for individuals who have demanding schedules.

• Stress Reduction: By focusing on areas prone to tension, such as the back, shoulders, and neck, chair massages can help reduce stress. Muscle tension release has the potential to enhance one's general state of relaxation.

• Enhanced Circulation: The implementation of massage techniques during chair massages has the potential to augment blood flow, thereby potentially enhancing systemic circulation.

• Muscle Tension Relief: By concentrating on high-risk areas susceptible to tension, such as the shoulders and neck, discomfort and rigidity in the muscles are alleviated.

• Enhanced Energy and Alertness: Certain individuals report heightened levels of energy and improved alertness subsequent to undergoing a chair massage, attributable to the prospective beneficial impacts that muscle relaxation may have on holistic health.

• Overall, massage has been linked to the secretion of endorphins, which are endogenous mood enhancers in the body. It is possible that chair massages could enhance one's disposition and sense of overall wellness.

• Physical distress may be mitigated for those who are seated at a desk or operating a computer for extended periods of time. By massaging the chair, problems associated with poor posture and prolonged seating can be remedied.

• Facilitates Relaxation: The calming ambiance and comfortable seating position provided by a chair massage contribute to the alleviation of tension and the promotion of relaxation.

- Chair massages are frequently more economical in cost than conventional full-body massages, thereby expanding their accessibility to a wider demographic.

It is imperative to acknowledge that personal experiences might differ, and although chair massages can offer a multitude of advantages, they might not be appropriate for all individuals. In addition, the proficiency and methodology employed by the massage therapist are factors that contribute to the overall efficacy of the massage.

Physiology And Anatomy Of Chair Massage

It is essential to comprehend the anatomy and physiology of the human body in order to perform chair massages effectively. The following are fundamental physiological and anatomical concepts pertinent to chair massage:

1. Muscular Structure:

• It is imperative to have knowledge of the main muscle groups, with particular emphasis on those located in the neck, shoulders, back, and arms. With this information, it is possible to target particular areas that are prone to stress and tension buildup.

• Muscle fiber trajectory is a crucial factor in facilitating the effective application of massage strokes.

2. Skeletal Structure:

• Understanding bony landmarks, including the spine, scapulae, and joints, is crucial for the massage therapist to effectively navigate the anatomy of the client and prevent the application of undue force to susceptible regions.

3. System of the Nervous System:

• Understanding nerve pathways and sensitive areas is crucial for modifying pressure and techniques in order to guarantee the comfort and safety of the client.

• Reflex points are areas where pressure is applied during chair massage; these points are associated with various bodily organs and systems.

4. Cardiovascular System:

• Blood Vessels: Knowledge of the location and pathways of blood vessels aids in the facilitation of blood flow and the avoidance of potential vascular trouble spots.

• Understanding the lymphatic system facilitates the promotion of lymphatic drainage and the reduction of fluid retention.

5. System of Integument (Skin):

• Skin Conditions: Maintaining knowledge of any skin conditions or sensitivities enables the massage therapist to modify techniques appropriately and select appropriate products.

6. The respiratory system consists of:

• Understanding the impact of breathing patterns on muscle tension enables the practitioner to facilitate clients' relaxation and promote deeper respiration throughout the massage.

7. Associative Tissues:

• The comprehension of the function of fascia, which is to connect and provide support for muscles and other structures, enables the development of massage techniques that target fascial restrictions.

8. Mobility and Range of Motion of the Joints:

• An understanding of the structure and function of joints is crucial in order to evaluate and improve joint mobility while performing massage techniques.

• The comprehension of the typical range of motion for joints is crucial for identifying any limitations and adjusting massage techniques accordingly.

9. Regarding Ergonomics and Posture:

• Postural Assessment: The evaluation of the client's posture serves the purpose of pinpointing specific areas of stress and devising a focused massage methodology.

• Ergonomics knowledge enables practitioners to provide clients with recommendations for posture enhancements and self-care techniques.

10. Responses of Physiology to Massage:

• Blood Pressure and Heart Rate: Understanding the potential impact of massage on these physiological parameters enables one to modify the massage's intensity.

• The comprehension of the potential endorphin release that

may occur during massage enhances the overall therapeutic impact.

Chair massage specialists in massage therapy should maintain an up-to-date understanding of anatomy and physiology in order to provide clients with safe and effective treatments that are specifically designed to their requirements.

CHAPTER TWO
Configuring A Chair Massage

Establishing the proper environment for chair massage is critical in order to provide a serene and comforting setting for the client and the massage therapist. Consider the following procedures when preparing a chair massage:

1. Select an Appropriate Location:

• Choose a secluded and tranquil location to guarantee the client's ease of mind and complete relaxation throughout the massage.

• When designing the space's illumination, strive to create a tranquil and calming atmosphere.

2. Choose an Appropriate Chair:

• Employ a specifically engineered massage chair that provides adequate body support for the client while facilitating the massage therapist's access.

• Ensure that clients of varying sizes can be accommodated by the chair's adjustability.

3. Organize the furnishings:

• Arrange the massage chair to facilitate unobstructed access for the massage therapist to the client's upper body, shoulders, back, and arms.

• Allocate sufficient space around the chair to accommodate the therapist's comfortable movement.

4. Implement Soft Cushions:

• To augment the client's comfort and support, particularly in regions such as the headrest and armrests, incorporate cushions or pillows.

5. Maintain Adequate Hygiene:

• It is essential to uphold a sanitary and pristine environment. Apply disposable coverings or recently laundered linens to the chair and any cushions.

• It is recommended to provide hand sanitizer to both the clinician and the client.

6. Define the Mood:

• To establish a tranquil ambiance, perform soothing, gentle music.

• To augment the sensory experience, contemplate incorporating essential oils or candles into aromatherapy settings.

7. Modify the Temperature by:

• Ensure the temperature of the room is suitable for comfort. If necessary, provide comforters or a shawl.

8. Engage in dialogue with the client:

• Inform the client of the chair massage procedure and what to anticipate throughout the session.

• Request any particular concerns or areas of emphasis that the client might possess.

9. Compose the Massage Equipment:

• Please ensure that massage oil, lotion, or ointment is easily accessible for the therapist to utilize throughout the massage.

• Maintain within easy reach any additional tools or accessories, including hot/cold compresses and massage tools.

10. Adopt a comfortable attire:

• It is recommended that both the client and the therapist don comfortable attire.

• During a chair massage, the client may remain completely clothed; therefore, clothing that is loose-fitting and easily removable is ideal.

11. Preserve Privacy:

• In order to establish a sense of privacy and guarantee the client's safety throughout the session, employ screens or draperies.

12. Deliver Post-Massage Solace:

• Provide clients with a designated area to rest and unwind following their massage.

• Provide the client with water or medicinal tea to aid in rehydration.

13. Instructions for Post:

• Deliver written or verbal directives regarding post-massage care, including but not limited to refraining from physically demanding activities and maintaining adequate hydration.

14. Preparing for Scheduling and Payment:

• Establish a system for payment and appointment scheduling, if applicable.

By diligently attending to these particulars, one can establish an environment that is both professional and conducive to chair massage, thereby enhancing the client's and therapist's experience.

Importance Of Tools And Supplies

It is essential to have the proper instruments and supplies when preparing for chair massage in order to guarantee a comfortable and effective experience. The following are indispensable equipment and materials for chair massage:

1. Chair with Massage Function:

• Invest in a high-quality, seated massage-specific adjustable massage chair. Ensure that it provides clients with adequate support and comfort.

2. Covers and linens:

• Inocent and comfortable linens or disposable chair coverings should be utilized to uphold hygiene standards and ensure that patrons have a pleasant experience.

3. Pillows and Cushions:

• One way to improve the comfort of the client is to incorporate supportive cushioning or pillows, focusing on areas such as the armrests and headrests.

4. Cream, Lotion, or Oil for Massage:

• To ensure the execution of effective and seamless massage strokes, select a massage oil, lotion, or crème of superior quality. Consider alternatives that emit calming aromas.

5. Sanitizing Spray or Wipes:

• Utilize sanitizing spray or wipes to sanitize the chair and any other client-touched surfaces prior to and following each session.

6. Towels consist of:

• Maintain a small towel supply for cleaning away excess lotion or oil and covering areas that are not undergoing a massage.

7. The use of aromatherapy:

• To enhance the overall massage experience and introduce calming fragrances, one may utilize essential oils, diffusers, or candles.

8. Sound and Speakers:

• To cultivate a tranquil atmosphere, initiate the playback of gentle, soothing music. Carry a portable speaker with you if the venue does not have audio equipment.

9. Hand Sanitizer consists of:

• It is recommended to provide hand disinfectant to both the massage therapist and the client in order to uphold personal hygiene.

10. Shawls or blankets:

• Distribute blankets or shawls to clients for warmth during the massage, particularly in chilly rooms.

11. Massage Equipment:

• To supplement manual techniques, consider utilizing additional massage instruments such as handheld massagers or percussion devices.

12. Cold/Hot Packs:

• Maintain a supply of heated or cold compresses to target particular areas of strain or discomfort.

13. The timer or clock:

• One should employ a timer or timepiece to monitor the progress of the massage session, guaranteeing that it adheres to the predetermined duration.

14. Items for Client Comfort:

• Provide supplementary comfort items, such as a neck support or eye pillow, in order to augment the client's state of relaxation.

15. Area for Post-Massage Comfort:

• Establish a designated area for patrons to recline and unwind subsequent to the massage, offering the option of water or herbal tea.

16. Forms of Massage Consent:

• Instruct clients to complete a concise consent form, which serves to verify their understanding of the massage's characteristics and any pertinent health considerations.

17. System for Payments and Scheduling:

• Establish a system for processing payments and scheduling future appointments, if applicable.

18. Cart or Portable Storage:

• Implement a portable cart or storage solution in order to maintain an orderly and accessible arrangement of your supplies.

By possessing these indispensable equipment and materials at your disposal, you will be adequately equipped to deliver a chair massage to your clientele that is both expertly executed and comfortable. Modify the assortment in accordance with the particular requirements of your clientele and the setting where you conduct chair massages.

CHAPTER THREE
Massage Techniques For Chairs

The purpose of chair massage techniques is to alleviate stress and stimulate relaxation in the client's upper body, shoulders, back, and limbs as they sit in an ergonomic chair. The following are frequent chair massage techniques:

1. Effleurage mechanisms:

• Utilize long, gliding palm and finger strokes to prepare the muscles for a more intense massage by warming them.

2. While kneading:

• By performing circular motions with the palms and fingertips, the muscles are lifted and kneaded. This improves circulation and aids in the discharge of tension.

3. The compression process:

• Implementing firm pressure on particular anatomical locations on the muscles using the hands, fingertips, or elbows. This may facilitate the discharge of tension and encourage relaxation.

4. Tapotement:

• Percussion or rhythmic tapping executed with the hands cupped, fists, or fingertips. This method has the potential to stimulate muscle activity and enhance blood flow.

5. The frictional force:

• For the purpose of targeting deeper layers of muscle tissue, employ circular or transverse motions with the thumbs or fingertips. This may assist in dissolving adhesions and knots.

6. The stretch:

• By performing light stretching exercises on the shoulders, back, neck, and arms, one can enhance flexibility and alleviate tension.

7. Point-of-trigger therapy:

• By directing concentrated pressure towards particular trigger points or knots in the musculature, one can alleviate localized tension.

8. Release of the Myofascial Tissue:

• The fascia (connective tissue) is subjected to sustained, gentle pressure in order to alleviate restrictions and enhance range of motion.

9. Fibre-crossed massage:

• Utilizing pressure applied perpendicular to the muscle fibers in order to increase flexibility and address adhesions.

10. Joint Activation:

• The implementation of low-impact exercises targets the joints' range of motion, with a particular emphasis on the shoulders, arms, and neck.

11. Pressure Acupoints:

• Pressure is applied to particular acupressure points in order to facilitate energy circulation and alleviate stress.

12. Neck Relaxation:

• Perform light neck rotations and stretches to alleviate tension and enhance mobility.

13. Shoulder Squeeze Motion:

• By employing a squeezing motion with the palms or fingertips on the shoulders, one can alleviate tightness in this prevalent area of tension.

14. Wrist and Forearm Massage:

• Particular attention should be paid to the forearms and wrists, particularly by those who engage in prolonged typing or computer usage.

15. Muscle Scapular Mobilization:

• By performing shoulder blade mobilization, one can alleviate tension and rigidity in the upper back.

16. Breathing Methods:

• Performing deep breathing exercises in order to promote a state of calm and relaxation.

17. Rocking Actions:

• Soft rocking or swaying motions can be utilized to promote muscle relaxation and alleviate spasming.

It is essential to customize chair massage techniques according to the client's specific requirements and preferences.

Effectively communicating with the client regarding their desired pressure, comfort level, and any specific areas of concern is essential for delivering a chair massage that is both enjoyable and productive.

Moreover, the maintenance of a consistent flow and cadence

throughout the massage session enhances its overall seamlessness and tranquility.

Safety Considerations And Contraindications

Although chair massage is generally regarded as safe and well-tolerated, massage therapists must be cognizant of specific contraindications and safety protocols to safeguard their clients.

Contraindications refer to specific conditions or circumstances that render massage unsuitable or potentially hazardous. Common chair massage contraindications and safety precautions are as follows:

Avoidance of contraindications:

1. Contagious Skin Disorders:

• Prevent the transmission of infections by refraining from massaging areas affected by exposed wounds, rashes, or contagious skin conditions.

2. Acquired Fever or Illness:

• It is advisable to delay the massage if the client is afflicted with an acute illness or has a fever, in order to prevent the transmission of the illness and permit the body to recuperate.

3. Recent Surgeries or Injuries:

• It is not advisable to massage areas that have recently undergone surgeries, fractures, or injuries without obtaining appropriate medical clearance.

4. Elevated Blood Pressure:

• It is imperative to exercise prudence and secure medical clearance prior to administering massage therapy to individuals whose hypertension is uncontrolled.

5. Risk of thrombosis or blood clots:

• It is not advisable for individuals with a prior medical history of thrombosis or blood clotting to engage in massage therapy on affected areas.

6. Recent Awakening:

• Before administering a massage to a client who has recently undergone traumatic events, such as a car accident, it is prudent to seek guidance from a healthcare professional.

7. Obstetric Complications:

• It is not advisable to massage expectant individuals who have preeclampsia, a history of preterm labor, or other complications without first consulting their healthcare provider.

8. Intense Pain:

• When massaging individuals who are in a critical state of pain, exercise prudence and seek guidance from a healthcare professional as necessary.

9. Inflammatory Disorders:

• Acutely inflamed areas, such as those experiencing flare-ups of rheumatoid arthritis, should not be massaged.

10. The Cancer Virus:

• Before receiving a massage, individuals undergoing cancer

treatment, particularly radiation or chemotherapy, should obtain clearance from their healthcare team.

Safety Precautions:

1. The Consultation with the Client:

• Preceding the massage, perform an extensive consultation to collect pertinent details regarding the client's medical background, present medications, and any particular apprehensions.

2. The Art of Communication:

• During the session, maintain an open line of communication with the client and encourage them to provide feedback regarding any discomfort, pressure, or comfort they may be experiencing.

3. Adjustment Methods:

• Incorporate modifications to massage techniques in accordance with the client's health status and level of comfort.

4. Hygiene Procedures:

• Adhere to appropriate hygiene protocols, which encompass handwashing and employing hand disinfectant, in order to avert the transmission of pathogens.

5. Honoring Boundaries:

• It is imperative to demonstrate adherence to the client's boundaries and preferences with respect to the specific areas that require massage. Assure that they are at ease and in charge throughout the session.

6. Ongoing Education and Accreditation:

• Maintain current training and certification in order to guarantee expertise in the most recent massage techniques and safety protocols.

7. Prepareness for Emergencies:

• Prepare oneself to address unforeseen circumstances, such as an abrupt illness or injury, through the implementation of an emergency plan.

8. After-Massage Care Guidelines:

• Please ensure to furnish comprehensive post-massage care guidelines that encompass proper hydration and specific activities to refrain from.

Massage therapists ought to consistently exercise their professional discretion and, in situations where uncertainty arises, seek advice from healthcare professionals regarding the suitability of massage for a specific client.

CHAPTER FOUR
Education And Communication
With Clients

Facilitating effective client education and communication are essential elements in delivering a successful chair massage experience.

Effective communication is essential for establishing trust, comprehending the requirements of the client, and guaranteeing the client's comfort and awareness. Critical elements of client education and communication in the context of chair massage are as follows.

1. Preliminary Consultation:

• Initiate every session with a concise consultation wherein the client's health history, particular concerns, and massage preferences are reviewed.

2. Consent by Informed Parties:

• Prior to commencing the chair massage session, obtain the client's informed consent and provide a thorough explanation of its nature. Specify the areas that will be targeted during the massage as well as any potential advantages or disadvantages.

3. Convenience for Clients:

• Maintain regular communication with the client to verify their comfort throughout the massage. Motivate them to express their inclinations concerning anxiety levels, areas of concentration, and any unease they might be experiencing.

4. Transmission of Methods:

• Explanation of the intended massage techniques and their potential benefits for the client in a concise manner. This can facilitate expectation management and guarantee that the client is cognizant of the therapeutic intent behind every technique.

5. Regarding feedback:

• Solicit feedback from the client both during and subsequent to the massage session. This may encompass evaluations regarding the level of pressure exerted, any specific areas of unease encountered, and the overall experience.

6. A personalized touch:

• Emphasize the capability of tailoring the massage to suit the particular requirements and inclinations of the client. Please elaborate on any particular areas of tension that they would like you to direct your attention towards.

7. Instruction Regarding Self-Care:

• Provide concise recommendations for self-care, including relaxation techniques and stretching routines, that patrons may integrate into their everyday schedules to enhance the therapeutic effects of the massage.

8. Safety and Hygiene Procedures:

• Disseminate the hygiene protocols that you adhere to, including handwashing and sanitization, in order to safeguard the welfare and security of the client.

9. Inform regarding Post-Massage Care:

• Deliver explicit post-massage care guidelines, encompassing recommendations for hydration, refraining from physically demanding activities, and any other pertinent maintenance suggestions.

10. Encourage Open Communication:

• Foster an environment that is transparent and impartial, encouraging clients to freely express their concerns, inquiries, or requirements.

11. Responding to Questions:

• Be ready to respond to the client's inquiries regarding the massage procedure, techniques, or overall well-being.

12. Establishing Practical Expectations:

• Effectively managing client expectations can be achieved through the provision of accurate and practical information pertaining to the potential advantages of chair massage, the length of time that relief lasts, and the significance of continuous self-care.

13. Post-Massage Deliberation:

• Engage in a post-massage conversation with the client to inquire about their emotional state, attend to any apprehensions, and offer suggestions for subsequent sessions or self-care routines.

14. Subsequent Communication:

• It is advisable to conduct post-session follow-up with clients, if applicable, to inquire about their welfare and motivate them to arrange subsequent appointments.

The establishment of a constructive client-therapist relationship is facilitated by open and honest communication, which also enhances the effectiveness and satisfaction of chair massage.

Adapt your approach to communication to suit the unique requirements and inclinations of every client, guaranteeing that they feel esteemed and adequately informed during the entirety of the procedure.

The Importance Of Chair Massage Practitioner Self-Care

It is imperative that chair massage practitioners practice self-care in order to preserve their physical and mental health, avert exhaustion, and ensure a lengthy and gratifying profession. The following are some self-care practices that practitioners of chair massage may wish to integrate into their daily regimen:

Physical Wellness:

1. Correct Physical Mechanics:

• To prevent strain, maintain proper body mechanics during massage appointments. Employ correct body alignment, maintain a balanced stance, and engage your core.

2. Consistent Stretching:

• Engage in consistent stretching routines to maintain muscular flexibility and alleviate tension. Concentrate on problem areas that are frequently targeted during massage therapy, including the neck, shoulders, and wrists.

3. Strength Conditioning:

• Enhance muscular strength in the upper body and core to promote proper posture and alleviate the physical strain experienced during massage sessions.

4. Consistent Exercise:

• Consistently participating in cardiovascular exercise will improve one's overall fitness and stamina. This may facilitate enhanced tension management and improved energy levels.

5. Consistent massages:

• It is advisable to establish a routine for receiving massages in order to reap the therapeutic advantages and alleviate any muscle tension or distress.

Emotional and mental self-care:

1. Zen-practice and meditation:

• Engaging in mindfulness or meditation can be beneficial for tension reduction, focus enhancement, and the maintenance of a tranquil and centered state of mind.

2. Developing Limitations:

• Isolate distinct parameters from clients and devise a timetable that accommodates sufficient periods of solitude and personal development.

3. Reflective Methods:

• Engage in introspection to evaluate your professional aspirations, accomplishments, and opportunities for development. This may foster a feeling of fulfillment and purpose.

4. Persisting in Education:

• Continue your pursuit of education in order to increase your expertise and understanding. This can maintain the vitality and freshness of your practice.

5. A harmonious work-life balance:

• To prevent exhaustion, maintain a healthy balance between work and personal life. Make time for leisure activities, personal interests, and quality time with loved ones.

Ergonomic Factors to Consider:

1. Superior Equipment:

• To support your practice, purchase high-quality massage instruments, including an adjustable and comfortable chair.

2. An Ergonomic Workplace Establishment:

- Establishing an ergonomic work environment that discourages physical strain and encourages proper posture is essential.

3. Consistent Breaks:

- Irrespective of the massage session, take frequent pauses to re-energize. During this period, extend, rehydrate, and unwind.

Emotional Assistance:

1. Peer Relationships:

- Establishing connections with fellow massage practitioners can provide support and the opportunity to share experiences. Peer connections can offer significant perspectives and provide emotional solace.

2. The provision of supervision or counseling:

• It is advisable to contemplate the utilization of professional supervision or counseling as a means to confront any emotional difficulties that may manifest within the course of your practice.

Workplace Conditions:

1.   **Articles   of   comfortable clothing:**

• To optimize one's physical comfort during massage appointments, it is advisable to don clothing that is both comfortable and supportive.

2. At ease in the workplace:

• Establish an inviting and pleasant work environment that fosters a positive and tranquil ambiance.

Routine Health Examinations:

1. Physical Health Observation:

• In order to effectively monitor one's overall physical health and promptly resolve any emerging issues, it is advisable to establish a routine for health check-ups.

2. Optical Care:

• Opt for proper eye hygiene, as prolonged periods of concentration during massages may cause ocular strain. Adhere to the 20-20-20 rule: observe an object at a distance of 20 feet for a minimum of 20 seconds every 20 minutes.

Time Administration:

1. Successful Scheduling:

• To prevent exhaustion, devise an efficient scheduling system that incorporates intervals for rest, vacations, and breaks.

2. Stress Administration:

• One potential strategy for managing tension in the workplace is to employ stress management techniques, such as progressive muscle relaxation or deep breathing exercises.

The state of financial well-being:

1. Financial strategizing:

• To alleviate the tension associated with financial uncertainties, it is advisable to execute prudent financial planning. This may involve strategies for financing, investing, and saving.

2. Coverage under Insurance:

• It is imperative to maintain adequate insurance coverage, including liability insurance, in order to safeguard one's professional interests.

Continuing Education and Development of Skills:

1. Advancements in Professional Development:

• Continuous professional development is essential for remaining up-to-date with industry trends and improving one's skill set.

2. Diversification of Skills:

• It is advisable to broaden one's repertoire of skills by delving into additional massage modalities or complementary therapies.

Various Relaxation Methods:

1. Breathing deeply exercises:

• Engage in deep breathing exercises as a means to alleviate tension and calm the nervous system.

2. Interests and Recreational Activities:

• Participate in extracurricular interests and recreational pursuits to restore one's mental and emotional well-being.

Bear in mind that self-care does not conform to a universal definition. It is critical to customize these practices to align with one's specific requirements, inclinations, and way of life. Consistent self-care not only yields individual advantages but also exerts a positive impact on the caliber of care one delivers to clients.

Summary

A multifaceted and easily obtainable modality of physical therapy, chair massage provides an abundance of advantages for practitioners and clients alike.

Prioritizing communication, safety, and self-care is equally as important as mastering effective massage techniques as it is to establish a prosperous chair massage practice.

Effective communication is crucial for practitioners as it fosters confidence and guarantees that clients are adequately informed regarding the massage procedure, methods, and possible results.

In addition, it permits a collaborative approach in which the massage therapist can customize the session according to the client's particular requirements and preferences.

Safety is of the utmost importance; therefore, practitioners must have an exhaustive knowledge of anatomy, contraindications, and hygiene procedures.

By abiding by established safety protocols, professionals have the ability to establish a safe and pleasant setting for their clientele.

The consideration and implementation of self-care practices are of equivalent significance for chair massage practitioners.

Consistent adherence to self-care practices, encompassing both physical and emotional well-being, is instrumental in ensuring the long-term viability of a massage profession. This includes balancing one's personal and professional life, managing stress, and maintaining good health.

Chair massage, due to its emphasis on convenience and abbreviated durations, is highly compatible with a wide range of environments, such as workplaces, gatherings, and public areas.

By incorporating strategies for effective communication, ensuring safety, and practicing self-care, practitioners of chair massage have the ability to generate a constructive and memorable encounter for their customers while simultaneously promoting their own vitality.

In the ever-evolving domain of massage therapy, continuous education and adjustment are imperative.

By remaining updated on industry trends, participating in ongoing education, and maintaining a receptive attitude towards evolving practices, practitioners actively contribute to the development and progression of chair massage as an invaluable therapeutic modality.

In general, chair massage serves as evidence of the efficacy of tactile stimulation in fostering relaxation, alleviating stress, and augmenting overall health and wellness within a variety of dynamic settings.

THE END

www.ingramcontent.com/pod-product-compliance
Lightning Source LLC
Chambersburg PA
CBHW050743260726
48661CB00001B/382